MACRO DIET COOKBOOK

FOR

BEGINNERS

Discover the Art of Macronutrient-Based Eating for Optimal Health, Weight Management, and Culinary Delight

by

Dr. Tracey Brannon

Table of Contents

Introduction

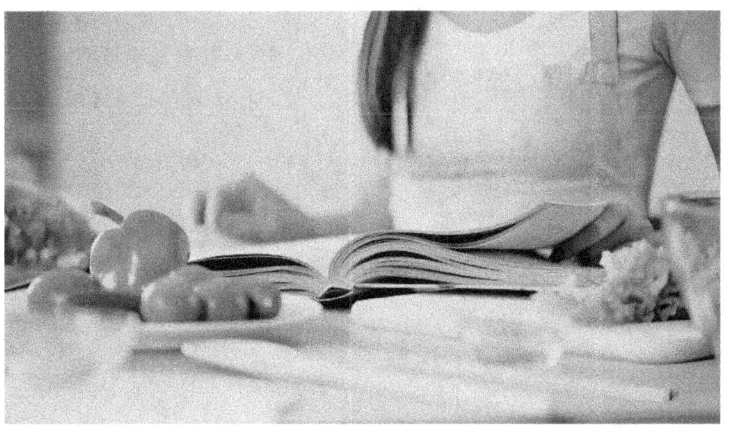

With the support of a Macro Diet Cookbook for Beginners, Emily set out on a path towards a healthy living in the midst of a busy city where fast food temptations were at every turn. Her eyes were opened to a universe of well-rounded eating as she turned the pages. She learned the basics of macronutrients and found a road map for making healthy, tasty meals in the cookbook.

Now that she knew more, Emily realized how important it was to be exact with her nutrition. She revamped her cooking routine chapter by chapter, discovering how to get the right amount of protein, carbs, and fats to fuel her day. The foods in the cookbook weren't simply a compilation of recipes; they were a path to a fuller, more fulfilling life. She got her day began with protein-packed breakfasts and kept going strong with balanced lunches.

The creative process of preparing brought satisfaction to Emily as she explored the many supper alternatives. As a result, snacks were useful tools for reducing bad urges, and the satisfying conclusions demonstrated that snacking need not be fraught with shame. Emily not only reached her health objectives but also found the deep joy of fueling her body with flavor and precision with the help of the Macro Diet Cookbook. The cookbook became her compass, steering her towards a path of wellbeing, one delicious meal at a time.

Macro Dieting

Macro dieting, short for macronutrient dieting, is a nutritional approach that focuses on the consumption of certain proportions of macronutrients—proteins, carbs, and fats—to attain health and fitness goals. Unlike typical diets that often concentrate calorie monitoring alone, macro dieting dives deeper into the quality and distribution of these critical nutrients.

At its foundation, macro dieting is about knowing the body's need for different macronutrients and adjusting one's diet accordingly. Proteins, the building blocks of muscles, play a critical function in recuperation and growth. Carbohydrates give energy, supporting physical activities and brain function. Fats, frequently misunderstood, contribute to hormone production and overall cellular function. The trick is in striking a balance adapted to individual needs, considering criteria such as age, activity level, and health objectives.

Embarking on a macro dieting journey needs a shift from perceiving food only as a source of calories to recognizing it as a giver of critical nutrients. This paradigm shift is liberating, as individuals acquire control over their nutritional intake, paving the door for sustained lifestyle adjustments.

Understanding Macronutrients

In the complicated fabric of nutrition, macronutrients form the backbone, performing key roles in sustaining life, supporting body functions, and impacting general health. Proteins, carbs, and fats are the trio that make up these macronutrients, each contributing distinctively to the body's welfare.

Proteins, sometimes touted as the body's building blocks, are important for growth, healing, and maintenance. Comprising amino acids, proteins serve as the structural underpinning for muscles, tissues, enzymes, and hormones. From lean meats and legumes to dairy products and plant-based sources, adopting a variety of protein-rich foods ensures a broad amino acid profile, needed for good health.

Carbohydrates, the body's major energy source, are classified into simple and complicated types. Simple carbohydrates, present in fruits and refined sugars, offer rapid energy bursts, while complex carbs, common in whole grains and vegetables, provide continuous energy. Understanding the glycemic index and eating carbs carefully assists individuals to manage blood sugar levels and sustain energy throughout the day.

Fats, often misunderstood, are necessary for different biological activities. Beyond being an energy reserve, lipids aid in nutrient absorption, promote brain health, and contribute to hormone production. Distinguishing between saturated and unsaturated fats and including sources like avocados, almonds, and olive oil ensures a balanced fat intake that promotes well-rounded health.

Achieving an ideal balance of these macronutrients is crucial to fulfilling individual health and fitness goals. The relevance of each macronutrient extends beyond its caloric content; it rests in the synergy between them. Macro dieting involves customizing the consumption of proteins, carbs, and fats to meet human needs, considering characteristics such as activity level, metabolism, and body composition.

Setting Your Macro Goals

In the domain of macro dieting, one size surely does not fit all. The beauty of this nutritional strategy resides in its adaptability, allowing individuals to modify their macronutrient consumption to correspond with their specific goals, lifestyles, and physiological needs. Setting macro goals becomes a cornerstone of this personalized path, requiring a mindful balance that goes beyond simply caloric concerns.

Understanding Individual Needs

Macro goals are not a onetime prescription but an evolving blueprint. Factors such as age, gender, exercise level, and overall health must be taken into account while developing personalized macro-objectives. A sedentary office worker, for instance, will have different requirements than an athlete engaging in hard training sessions. Recognizing the changing nature of these demands lays the way for a more effective and sustainable approach to macro goalsetting.

Caloric Considerations and Macronutrient Ratios

While calories count, macro dieting goes beyond the simple arithmetic of intake vs expenditure. It concentrates emphasis on the distribution of macronutrients in the total caloric profile. Protein, frequently valued for its musclebuilding characteristics, may be raised for those focusing on strength exercise. Carbohydrate intake may be altered based on energy demands, and lipids may be modulated to meet certain health objectives.

Balancing Act for Health and Fitness

Setting macro goals is a complex balancing act, akin to composing a tailored symphony of nutrients. Achieving the appropriate balance ensures energy sustainability, muscle preservation, and metabolic optimization. It also plays a critical part in weight control, whether the aim is fat loss, muscle gain, or simply maintaining a healthy body composition.

Tools and Tracking

To embark on this journey, adopting tools such as macro calculators and tracking applications becomes important. These tools assist measure macronutrient demands, track food intake, and analyze progress. While precision is beneficial, flexibility is also vital. Macro goals should act as guiding principles rather than rigid constraints, giving opportunity for lifestyle variances and unforeseen occurrences.

Evaluating and Adjusting

Macro goals are not set in stone. Regular appraisals of progress and modifications to the macronutrient profile are crucial to ongoing success. Adapting to variations in activity levels, responding to alterations in weight, and accepting developing fitness goals all demand periodic appraisal and recalibration of macro targets.

Essential Kitchen Tools and Ingredients for Macro Cooking

Embarking on a journey into macro cuisine involves not just knowledge of macronutrients but also a well-equipped kitchen ready to translate that information into culinary pleasures. As you set the stage for your macro-based culinary expedition, consider the crucial tools and ingredients that will convert your kitchen into a hub of balanced, delectable, and health-conscious meals.

Kitchen Tools

1. Food Scale

A food scale becomes your trusted ally for accurate portion management, a cornerstone of macro dieting. Accurate measurements of components guarantee that you reach your macronutrient objectives with precision.

2. Measuring Cups and Spoons

These culinary essentials are crucial for measuring items including grains, liquids, and oils. Consistency in measures is crucial to keeping the proper macronutrient ratios in your meals.

3. Blender or Food Processor

These multipurpose tools are important for preparing smoothies, sauces, and dips. They allow you to combine diverse macro-friendly products into delicious and nutritious creations.

4. Quality Cookware

Invest in high-quality pots, pans, and baking sheets to ensure consistent cooking and minimize sticking. Nonstick surfaces eliminate the need for unnecessary cooking oils, helping you control your fat intake.

5. Meal Prep Containers

Portion management and planning are at the foundation of macro cooking. Durable, stackable containers promote fast meal planning, making it easier to stay on track with your dietary goals.

Macro-Friendly Ingredients

1. Lean Proteins

Incorporate lean protein sources such as chicken breast, turkey, fish, tofu, and lentils. These alternatives are rich in protein, promoting muscle maintenance and growth.

2. Whole Grains

Opt for complex carbohydrates like brown rice, quinoa, oats, and whole wheat pasta. These grains give lasting energy, keeping you fed throughout the day.

3. Healthy Fats

Include sources of healthy fats including avocados, nuts, seeds, and olive oil. These fats contribute to general wellbeing and add depth to your meals without compromising on nutritional goals.

4. Colorful Vegetables

Load up on a variety of colorful veggies to provide a wide range of vitamins, minerals, and antioxidants. These low-calorie, high-nutrient options are crucial to a well-rounded macro-focused diet.

5. Low-Glycemic Fruits

Opt for fruits that are lower on the glycemic index, such as berries, apples, and citrus fruits. These selections deliver natural sweetness without producing abrupt rises in blood sugar levels.

6. Herbs and Spices

Elevate the flavor of your macro meals with a choice of herbs and spices. Not only can they offer dimension to your recipes, but many also come with their own set of health advantages.

As you prepare your kitchen arsenal, remember that macro cooking is not just about reaching nutritional goals—it's a culinary journey that embraces the interplay of flavors and nourishment. Armed with the correct tools and resources, your kitchen becomes a canvas for designing meals that are both delicious and connected with your macro path.

Benefits of Macro Diet

The Macro Diet, also known as flexible dieting, has achieved considerable popularity because to its emphasis on balance, customization, and sustainable nutrition. This strategy emphasizes on the consumption of macronutrients—proteins, carbs, and fats—allowing individuals to achieve their nutritional needs while enjoying a variety of meals. The benefits of the Macro Diet extend far beyond weight management, embracing general health and wellbeing.

One of the primary advantages of the Macro Diet is its versatility. Unlike restrictive diets that impose certain food choices, the Macro Diet gives freedom in selecting meals that match with individual preferences and nutritional requirements. This flexibility not only promotes adherence but also encourages a good relationship with food, encouraging long-term success.

A significant component of the Macro Diet is its capacity to support diverse fitness goals. Whether someone seeks to lose weight, grow muscle, or maintain general health, the adjustable aspect of macro tracking enables individuals to adapt their nutritional consumption accordingly. Athletes, fitness enthusiasts, and those involved in specific training programs find the Macro Diet essential in boosting their performance and recovery.

Balancing macronutrients aids to consistent energy levels throughout the day. Properly divided protein, carbs, and fats offer a steady release of energy, eliminating spikes and crashes that commonly follow diets high in simple sugars. This continuous energy flow improves cognitive function, physical endurance, and general vitality.

Moreover, the Macro Diet encourages awareness of portion sizes and nutritional content. By measuring macros, individuals get a better grasp of the nutritional content of different foods, enabling educated decisions. This heightened awareness can lead to improved meal selection, making it easier to meet micronutrient demands and increase overall health.

The Macro Diet is not just focused on appearances; it stresses total health and well-rounded nourishment. Adequate protein consumption supports muscle maintenance and regeneration, essential for people engaging in physical activity or resistance training. Balanced carbs provide a sustainable source of energy, while healthy fats play a critical role in hormone production and absorption of fat-soluble vitamins.

This dietary approach is sustainable in the long run, as it doesn't identify things as totally off-limits. Instead, it emphasizes moderation and teaches individuals to integrate their favorite foods while staying within their macronutrient targets. This element decreases feelings of deprivation commonly associated with traditional dieting, encouraging a better perspective regarding food.

Furthermore, the Macro Diet can be altered to fit diverse dietary preferences, including vegetarian, vegan, or gluten-free lifestyles. This universality makes it accessible to a broad spectrum of persons seeking a personalized and effective approach to nutrition.

Macro Diet distinguishes out for its adaptability, sustainability, and favorable influence on overall health. By emphasizing the significance of macronutrient balance and giving flexibility in food choices, this strategy encourages individuals to attain their fitness and wellness goals while enjoying a diversified and delicious diet.

Chapter 1: Breakfast Recipes

Protein-Packed Omelette

Prep Time:10 minutes

Ingredients:

- 3 eggs
- 1/2 cup diced bell peppers
- 1/4 cup diced onions
- 1/4 cup diced tomatoes
- 1/4 cup shredded low-fat cheese

Instructions:

- Whisk eggs in a bowl and pour into a hot, nonstick skillet.
- Add vegetables and cheese.
- Cook until the edges are set, then fold the omelette.

Nutritional Value:

- Protein: 25g
- Carbohydrates: 8g
- Fats: 12g

Greek Yogurt Parfait

Prep Time: 5 minutes

Ingredients:

- 1 cup Greek yogurt
- 1/2 cup mixed berries
- 1/4 cup granola
- Drizzle of honey

Instructions:

- Layer yogurt, berries, and granola in a glass.
- Repeat the layers.
- Drizzle with honey before serving.

Nutritional Value:

- Protein: 20g
- Carbohydrates: 30g
- Fats: 8g

Quinoa Breakfast Bowl

Prep Time: 15 minutes

Ingredients:

- 1/2 cup cooked quinoa
- 1/4 cup almond milk
- 1 tablespoon chia seeds
- Sliced banana and a handful of blueberries

Instructions:

- Mix quinoa with almond milk and chia seeds.
- Top with sliced banana and blueberries.

Nutritional Value:

- Protein: 10g
- Carbohydrates: 40g
- Fats: 5g

Whole Wheat Pancake

Prep Time: 20 minutes

Ingredients:

- 1 cup whole wheat flour
- 1 tablespoon baking powder
- 1 cup almond milk
- 1 egg

Instructions:

- Mix flour, baking powder, almond milk, and egg.
- Cook pancakes on a hot griddle.

Nutritional Value:

- Protein: 12g
- Carbohydrates: 30g
- Fats: 5g

Avocado Toast with Poached Eggs

Prep Time: 15 minutes

Ingredients:

- 2 slices whole grain bread
- 1 ripe avocado
- 2 poached eggs
- Salt and pepper to taste

Instructions:

- Mash avocado and spread it on toasted bread.
- Top with poached eggs and season.

Nutritional Value:

- Protein: 15g
- Carbohydrates: 20g
- Fats: 18g

Sweet Potato Breakfast Hash

Prep Time: 25 minutes

Ingredients:

- 1 sweet potato, diced
- 1/2 cup black beans
- 1/4 cup diced bell peppers
- 1/4 cup diced onions

Instructions:

- Roast sweet potatoes, then sauté with beans and vegetables.
- Cook until everything is tender.

Nutritional Value:

- Protein: 8g
- Carbohydrates: 35g
- Fats: 2g

Spinach and Feta Egg Muffins

Prep Time:15 minutes

Ingredients:

- 4 eggs
- 1 cup fresh spinach, chopped
- 1/4 cup crumbled feta cheese

Instructions:

- Whisk eggs, then mix with spinach and feta.
- Pour into muffin cups and bake until set.

Nutritional Value:

- Protein: 18g
- Carbohydrates: 2g
- Fats: 12g

Cottage Cheese and Fruit Bowl

Prep Time: 10 minutes

Ingredients:

- 1 cup low-fat cottage cheese
- 1/2 cup pineapple chunks
- 1/2 cup sliced strawberries

Instructions:

- Mix cottage cheese with fresh fruit.
- Serve chilled.

Nutritional Value:

- Protein: 25g
- Carbohydrates: 20g
- Fats: 5g

Egg White Veggie Scramble

Prep Time: 12 minutes

Ingredients:

- 1 cup egg whites
- 1/2 cup diced zucchini
- 1/4 cup diced tomatoes
- 1/4 cup chopped spinach

Instructions:

- Cook egg whites in a skillet, add veggies, and scramble.
- Season to taste.

Nutritional Value:

- Protein: 20g
- Carbohydrates: 5g
- Fats: 2g

Peanut Butter Banana Smoothie

Prep Time: 5 minutes

Ingredients:

- 1 banana
- 2 tablespoons peanut butter
- 1 cup almond milk
- Ice cubes (optional)

Instructions:

- Blend banana, peanut butter, and almond milk until smooth.
- Add ice cubes if desired.

Nutritional Value:

- Protein: 12g
- Carbohydrates: 30g
- Fats: 15g

These breakfast recipes not only cater to your macro needs but also infuse your mornings with energy, flavor, and a nutritional kickstart for the day ahead.

Chapter 2: Lunch Recipes

Grilled Chicken Quinoa Bowl

Prep Time: 20 minutes

Ingredients:

- 6 oz grilled chicken breast
- 1 cup cooked quinoa
- 1/2 cup roasted vegetables (zucchini, bell peppers)
- 1 tablespoon olive oil

Instructions:

- Combine grilled chicken, quinoa, and roasted vegetables.
- Drizzle with olive oil and toss gently.

Nutritional Value:

- Protein: 30g
- Carbohydrates: 40g

- Fats: 15g

Salmon and Asparagus Stir-Fry

Prep Time: 15 minutes

Ingredients:

- 8 oz salmon fillet, cubed
- 1 cup asparagus, sliced
- 1/4 cup soy sauce
- 1 tablespoon sesame oil

Instructions:

- Stir-fry salmon and asparagus in sesame oil.
- Add soy sauce and cook until salmon is done.

Nutritional Value:

- Protein: 25g
- Carbohydrates: 10g
- Fats: 15g

Quinoa and Black Bean Salad

Prep Time: 15 minutes

Ingredients:

- 1 cup cooked quinoa
- 1/2 cup black beans, drained
- 1/4 cup corn kernels
- 1/4 cup diced tomatoes

Instructions:

- Mix quinoa, black beans, corn, and tomatoes.
- Toss with your favorite vinaigrette.

Nutritional Value:

- Protein: 15g
- Carbohydrates: 35g
- Fats: 5g

Turkey and Veggie Wrap

Prep Time: 10 minutes

Ingredients:

- 4 oz turkey slices
- Whole grain wrap
- 1/2 cup lettuce, shredded
- 1/4 cup sliced cucumbers

Instructions:

- Lay turkey on the wrap, add lettuce and cucumbers.
- Roll up tightly and slice into halves.

Nutritional Value:

- Protein: 20g
- Carbohydrates: 30g
- Fats: 8g

Mediterranean Chickpea Salad

Prep Time: 15 minutes

Ingredients:

- 1 can chickpeas, drained
- 1/2 cup cherry tomatoes, halved
- 1/4 cup red onion, finely chopped
- Feta cheese crumbles

Instructions:

- Combine chickpeas, tomatoes, and red onion.
- Top with feta cheese and toss.

Nutritional Value:

- Protein: 12g
- Carbohydrates: 30g
- Fats: 10g

Vegetarian Quiche with Spinach and Mushrooms

Prep Time: 30 minutes

Ingredients:

- 4 eggs
- 1 cup spinach, chopped
- 1/2 cup mushrooms, sliced
- 1/4 cup feta cheese

Instructions:

- Whisk eggs, then mix with spinach, mushrooms, and feta.
- Pour into a pie dish and bake until set.

Nutritional Value:

- Protein: 15g
- Carbohydrates: 10g
- Fats: 12g

Shrimp and Quinoa Stir-Fry

Prep Time: 20 minutes

Ingredients:
- 8 oz shrimp, peeled and deveined
- 1 cup cooked quinoa
- 1/2 cup broccoli florets
- 1/4 cup soy sauce

Instructions:
- Stirfry shrimp and broccoli in soy sauce.
- Add cooked quinoa and toss until well combined.

Nutritional Value:
- Protein: 25g
- Carbohydrates: 30g
- Fats: 8g

Caprese Chicken Salad

Prep Time: 15 minutes

Ingredients:

- 6 oz grilled chicken breast
- 1 cup cherry tomatoes, halved
- Fresh mozzarella balls
- Fresh basil leaves

Instructions:

- Combine chicken, tomatoes, mozzarella, and basil.
- Drizzle with balsamic glaze before serving.

Nutritional Value:

- Protein: 30g
- Carbohydrates: 10g
- Fats: 15g

Lentil and Vegetable Soup

Prep Time: 25 minutes

Ingredients:

- 1 cup lentils, rinsed
- 1/2 cup carrots, diced
- 1/4 cup celery, chopped
- 1/4 cup onion, finely chopped

Instructions:

- Cook lentils with vegetables until tender.
- Season to taste and simmer until flavors meld.

Nutritional Value:

- Protein: 18g
- Carbohydrates: 40g
- Fats: 2g

Sesame Ginger Tofu Stir-Fry

Prep Time: 20 minutes

Ingredients:

- 1 cup tofu, cubed
- 1 cup mixed stir-fry vegetables
- 2 tablespoons soy sauce
- 1 tablespoon sesame oil

Instructions:

- Sauté tofu and vegetables in sesame oil.
- Add soy sauce and stir until wellcoated.

Nutritional Value:

- Protein: 15g
- Carbohydrates: 20g
- Fats: 10g

Chapter 3: Dinner Recipes

Grilled Salmon with Lemon Dill Sauce

Prep Time: 15 minutes

Ingredients:

- 8 oz salmon fillet
- 1 lemon (juiced)
- 1 tablespoon fresh dill, chopped
- Salt and pepper to taste

Instructions:

- Grill salmon, squeeze lemon juice over it, and sprinkle with dill.
- Season with salt and pepper before serving.

Nutritional Value:

- Protein: 30g
- Carbohydrates: 1g
- Fats: 15g

Quinoa Stuffed Bell Peppers

Prep Time: 30 minutes

Ingredients:

- 1 cup cooked quinoa

- 4 bell peppers, halved

- 1/2 cup black beans, drained

- 1/2 cup corn kernels

Instructions:

- Mix quinoa, black beans, and corn.

- Stuff bell peppers and bake until tender.

Nutritional Value:

- Protein: 12g

- Carbohydrates: 30g

- Fats: 5g

Chicken and Broccoli Stir-Fry

Prep Time: 20 minutes

Ingredients:

- 8 oz chicken breast, sliced
- 2 cups broccoli florets
- 1/4 cup soy sauce
- 1 tablespoon sesame oil

Instructions:

- Stir-fry chicken and broccoli in sesame oil.
- Add soy sauce and cook until chicken is done.

Nutritional Value:

- Protein: 25g
- Carbohydrates: 10g
- Fats: 12g

Eggplant and Chickpea Curry

Prep Time: 25 minutes

Ingredients:

- 1 large eggplant, diced
- 1 can chickpeas, drained
- 1 cup tomatoes, diced
- 2 tablespoons curry powder

Instructions:

- Sauté eggplant, add chickpeas, tomatoes, and curry powder.
- Simmer until eggplant is tender.

Nutritional Value:

- Protein: 10g
- Carbohydrates: 30g
- Fats: 5g

Turkey and Vegetable Skewers

Prep Time: 20 minutes

Ingredients:

- 8 oz turkey breast, cubed
- Cherry tomatoes
- Zucchini slices
- Red onion chunks

Instructions:

- Thread turkey and vegetables onto skewers.
- Grill until turkey is cooked through.

Nutritional Value:

- Protein: 25g
- Carbohydrates: 10g
- Fats: 8g

Sweet Potato and Black Bean Chili

Prep Time: 30 minutes

Ingredients:

- 2 sweet potatoes, diced
- 1 can black beans, drained
- 1 cup diced tomatoes
- 1 tablespoon chili powder

Instructions:

- Cook sweet potatoes, add black beans, tomatoes, and chili powder.
- Simmer until flavors meld.

Nutritional Value:

- Protein: 15g
- Carbohydrates: 40g
- Fats: 2g

Lemon Herb Grilled Chicken

Prep Time: 15 minutes

Ingredients:

- 6 oz chicken breast
- Zest and juice of 1 lemon
- 1 tablespoon mixed herbs (rosemary, thyme)
- Salt and pepper to taste

Instructions:

- Marinate chicken in lemon, herbs, salt, and pepper.
- Grill until cooked through.

Nutritional Value:

- Protein: 30g
- Carbohydrates: 1g
- Fats: 12g

Shrimp and Vegetable Stir-Fry

Prep Time: 20 minutes

Ingredients:

- 8 oz shrimp, peeled and deveined
- 2 cups mixed stir-fry vegetables
- 1/4 cup soy sauce
- 1 tablespoon sesame oil

Instructions:

- Stir-fry shrimp and vegetables in sesame oil.
- Add soy sauce and cook until shrimp is done.

Nutritional Value:

- Protein: 25g
- Carbohydrates: 15g
- Fats: 10g

Mushroom and Spinach Stuffed Chicken Breast

Prep Time: 30 minutes

Ingredients:

- 2 chicken breasts
- 1 cup mushrooms, chopped
- 1 cup fresh spinach
- 1/4 cup feta cheese

Instructions:

- Sauté mushrooms and spinach, stuff into chicken breasts with feta.
- Bake until chicken is cooked through.

Nutritional Value:

- Protein: 30g
- Carbohydrates: 5g
- Fats: 15g

Vegetarian Lentil Meatballs

Prep Time: 25 minutes

Ingredients:

- 1 cup cooked lentils
- 1/2 cup breadcrumbs
- 1/4 cup grated Parmesan cheese
- Marinara sauce for serving

Instructions:

- Mash lentils, mix with breadcrumbs and cheese.
- Form into meatballs and bake until golden.

Nutritional Value:

- Protein: 15g
- Carbohydrates: 25g
- Fats: 5g

These nourishing dinner recipes not only cater to diverse palates but also offer a wholesome balance of macronutrients to support your wellbeing.

Chapter 4: Snacks and Sides

Greek Yogurt and Berry Parfait

Prep Time: 5 minutes

Ingredients:

- 1 cup Greek yogurt
- Mixed berries (strawberries, blueberries)
- Granola
- Honey for drizzling

Instructions:

- Layer Greek yogurt, berries, and granola in a glass.
- Drizzle with honey. Serve chilled.

Nutritional Value:

- Protein: 15g
- Carbohydrates: 30g
- Fats: 8g

Hummus and Veggie Platter

Prep Time: 10 minutes

Ingredients:

- Hummus
- Carrot sticks, cucumber slices
- Cherry tomatoes
- Whole grain pita wedges

Instructions:

- Arrange veggies and pita around a bowl of hummus.
- Dip and enjoy this healthy and satisfying snack.

Nutritional Value:

- Protein: 8g
- Carbohydrates: 20g
- Fats: 10g

Caprese Skewers

Prep Time: 15 minutes

Ingredients:

- Cherry tomatoes
- Fresh mozzarella balls
- Basil leaves
- Balsamic glaze for drizzling

Instructions:

- Thread tomatoes, mozzarella, and basil onto skewers.
- Drizzle with balsamic glaze. Serve as a refreshing side.

Nutritional Value:

- Protein: 10g
- Carbohydrates: 5g
- Fats: 8g

Baked Sweet Potato Fries

Prep Time: 20 minutes

Ingredients:

- Sweet potatoes, cut into fries
- Olive oil
- Paprika, garlic powder
- Sea salt and black pepper

Instructions:

- Toss sweet potato fries in olive oil and seasonings.
- Bake until crispy. A nutritious alternative to regular fries.

Nutritional Value:

- Protein: 2g
- Carbohydrates: 30g
- Fats: 8g

Edamame and Sea Salt

Prep Time: 5 minutes

Ingredients:
- Edamame (steamed and cooled)
- Coarse sea salt

Instructions:
- Sprinkle edamame with sea salt. A simple and protein-rich snack.

Nutritional Value:
- Protein: 17g
- Carbohydrates: 15g
- Fats: 8g

Whole Grain Crackers with Tuna Salad

Prep Time: 10 minutes

Ingredients:

- Whole grain crackers
- Canned tuna, drained
- Greek yogurt
- Diced celery, red onion

Instructions:

- Mix tuna with Greek yogurt, celery, and onion.
- Spoon onto crackers. A balanced and satisfying snack.

Nutritional Value:

- Protein: 15g
- Carbohydrates: 20g
- Fats: 8g

Roasted Chickpeas

Prep Time: 15 minutes

Ingredients:

- Canned chickpeas, drained
- Olive oil
- Smoked paprika, cumin
- Salt and cayenne pepper

Instructions:

- Toss chickpeas in olive oil and seasonings.
- Roast until crispy. A crunchy and fiberrich snack.

Nutritional Value:

- Protein: 15g
- Carbohydrates: 30g
- Fats: 8g

Cucumber and Tzatziki Dip

Prep Time: 10 minutes

Ingredients:

- Cucumber, sliced
- Greek yogurt
- Garlic, dill
- Lemon juice

Instructions:

- Mix Greek yogurt with grated cucumber, garlic, dill, and lemon juice.
- Serve with cucumber slices. A cool and refreshing side.

Nutritional Value:

- Protein: 8g
- Carbohydrates: 10g
- Fats: 5g

Trail Mix with Nuts and Dried Fruit

Prep Time: 5 minutes

Ingredients:

- Almonds, walnuts, cashews
- Dried cranberries, raisins
- Dark chocolate chips

Instructions:

- Mix nuts, dried fruit, and chocolate chips.
- Portion into snacksized bags for a quick energy boost.

Nutritional Value:

- Protein: 10g
- Carbohydrates: 20g
- Fats: 15g

Avocado and Tomato Salsa

Prep Time: 10 minutes

Ingredients:

- Avocado, diced
- Tomatoes, diced
- Red onion, finely chopped
- Cilantro, lime juice

Instructions:

- Mix avocado, tomatoes, onion, cilantro, and lime juice.
- Serve with whole grain tortilla chips. A nutrient-packed dip.

Nutritional Value:

- Protein: 5g
- Carbohydrates: 15g
- Fats: 10g

These smart choices for snacks and sides not only satisfy your cravings but also provide a nutritional boost to enhance your daily wellbeing.

Chapter 5: Sweet Endings

Protein-Packed Chocolate Smoothie Bowl

Prep Time: 10 minutes

Ingredients:

- 1 scoop chocolate protein powder
- 1 frozen banana
- 1 cup unsweetened almond milk
- Toppings: sliced strawberries, chia seeds

Instructions:

- Blend protein powder, banana, and almond milk until smooth.
- Pour into a bowl, top with strawberries and chia seeds.

Nutritional Value:

- Protein: 25g
- Carbohydrates: 30g
- Fats: 8g

Baked Apples with Cinnamon

Prep Time: 20 minutes

Ingredients:

- 2 apples, cored and halved
- 1 teaspoon cinnamon
- 1 tablespoon honey
- Chopped nuts for garnish

Instructions:

- Preheat oven. Sprinkle apples with cinnamon, drizzle with honey.
- Bake until tender. Garnish with chopped nuts before serving.

Nutritional Value:

- Protein: 2g
- Carbohydrates: 30g
- Fats: 5g

Chia Seed Pudding with Berries

Prep Time: 5 minutes (+ chilling time)

Ingredients:

- 3 tablespoons chia seeds
- 1 cup almond milk
- Mixed berries
- 1 tablespoon maple syrup

Instructions:

- Mix chia seeds and almond milk. Refrigerate until set.
- Top with mixed berries and drizzle with maple syrup.

Nutritional Value:

- Protein: 10g
- Carbohydrates: 25g
- Fats: 8g

Frozen Banana Bites

Prep Time: 15 minutes (+ freezing time)

Ingredients:
- Bananas, sliced
- Greek yogurt
- Dark chocolate, melted
- Crushed nuts for coating

Instructions:
- Dip banana slices in yogurt, then chocolate, and coat with nuts.
- Freeze until solid. A delightful and guiltfree frozen treat.

Nutritional Value:
- Protein: 5g
- Carbohydrates: 20g
- Fats: 10g

Avocado Chocolate Mousse

Prep Time: 10 minutes

Ingredients:

- 2 ripe avocados
- 1/4 cup cocoa powder
- 1/4 cup maple syrup
- Vanilla extract

Instructions:

- Blend avocados, cocoa powder, maple syrup, and vanilla until smooth.
- Chill before serving. A creamy and indulgent dessert.

Nutritional Value:

- Protein: 5g
- Carbohydrates: 25g
- Fats: 15g

Coconut and Almond Energy Bites

Prep Time: 15 minutes (+ chilling time)

Ingredients:

- 1 cup rolled oats
- 1/2 cup almond butter
- 1/4 cup honey
- Shredded coconut for rolling

Instructions:

- Mix oats, almond butter, and honey. Form into bitesized balls.
- Roll in shredded coconut. Refrigerate until firm.

Nutritional Value:

- Protein: 8g
- Carbohydrates: 20g
- Fats: 12g

Berry and Yogurt Parfait

Prep Time: 10 minutes

Ingredients:
- Mixed berries
- Greek yogurt
- Granola
- Drizzle of honey

Instructions:
- Layer berries, yogurt, and granola in a glass.
- Repeat layers. Drizzle with honey. A delightful and wholesome dessert.

Nutritional Value:
- Protein: 10g
- Carbohydrates: 30g
- Fats: 8g

Peanut Butter Banana Oat Cookies

Prep Time: 20 minutes

Ingredients:

- 2 ripe bananas, mashed
- 1 cup rolled oats
- 1/4 cup peanut butter
- Dark chocolate chips (optional)

Instructions:

- Mix mashed bananas, oats, and peanut butter.
- Drop spoonfuls onto a baking sheet. Bake until golden.

Nutritional Value:

- Protein: 6g
- Carbohydrates: 25g
- Fats: 10g

Cinnamon Vanilla Rice Pudding

Prep Time: 30 minutes

Ingredients:

- 1 cup Arborio rice
- 4 cups almond milk
- 1/4 cup maple syrup
- Cinnamon and vanilla extract

Instructions:

- Cook rice in almond milk until creamy. Stir in maple syrup.
- Add cinnamon and vanilla to taste. A comforting and sweet ending.

Nutritional Value:

- Protein: 5g
- Carbohydrates: 30g
- Fats: 8g

Mango Sorbet

Prep Time: 5 minutes (+ freezing time)

Ingredients:

- Frozen mango chunks
- 1/4 cup coconut water
- Fresh mint leaves for garnish

Instructions:

- Blend frozen mango with coconut water until smooth.
- Freeze until firm. Garnish with fresh mint before serving.

Nutritional Value:

- Protein: 2g
- Carbohydrates: 25g
- Fats: 1g

These macrofriendly desserts offer a sweet ending without compromising your nutritional goals, providing a guiltfree treat for your taste buds.

Chapter 6: Chicken and Turkey

Grilled Lemon Herb Chicken Breast

Prep Time: 15 minutes

Ingredients:

- 4 boneless, skinless chicken breasts
- Zest and juice of 2 lemons
- Mixed herbs (rosemary, thyme)
- Salt and pepper to taste

Instructions:

- Marinate chicken in lemon zest, juice, herbs, salt, and pepper.
- Grill until fully cooked. Serve with steamed vegetables.

Nutritional Value:

- Protein: 30g
- Carbohydrates: 1g
- Fats: 12g

Turkey and Quinoa Stuffed Peppers

Prep Time: 30 minutes

Ingredients:

- 1 lb ground turkey
- 1 cup cooked quinoa
- Bell peppers (various colors)
- Tomato sauce

Instructions:

- Brown turkey, mix with cooked quinoa.
- Stuff bell peppers, top with tomato sauce. Bake until peppers are tender.

Nutritional Value:

- Protein: 25g
- Carbohydrates: 30g
- Fats: 8g

Baked Pesto Chicken Thighs

Prep Time: 20 minutes

Ingredients:

- 8 chicken thighs, bonein, skinon
- 1/2 cup basil pesto
- Garlic powder, salt, and pepper

Instructions:

- Preheat oven. Rub chicken with pesto, season with garlic, salt, and pepper.
- Bake until golden and cooked through. Serve with a side salad.

Nutritional Value:

- Protein: 30g
- Carbohydrates: 2g
- Fats: 20g

Turkey and Vegetable Stir-Fry

Prep Time: 20 minutes

Ingredients:

- 1 lb turkey breast, thinly sliced
- Mixed stir-fry vegetables (broccoli, bell peppers, snap peas)
- Soy sauce, ginger, and garlic

Instructions:

- Stir-fry turkey and vegetables in a pan with soy sauce, ginger, and garlic.
- Cook until turkey is done. Serve over brown rice or quinoa.

Nutritional Value:

- Protein: 25g
- Carbohydrates: 15g
- Fats: 8g

Chicken and Spinach Stuffed Portobello Mushrooms

Prep Time: 25 minutes

Ingredients:

- 4 large portobello mushrooms
- 1 lb ground chicken
- Fresh spinach, garlic, and onion
- Feta cheese (optional)

Instructions:

- Sauté chicken with spinach, garlic, and onion.
- Stuff mushrooms, bake until mushrooms are tender. Top with feta if desired.

Nutritional Value:

- Protein: 25g
- Carbohydrates: 5g
- Fats: 15g

Turkey and Sweet Potato Skillet

Prep Time: 30 minutes

Ingredients:

- 1 lb ground turkey
- Sweet potatoes, diced
- Onion, bell peppers, and garlic
- Taco seasoning

Instructions:

- Brown turkey, add diced sweet potatoes, vegetables, and taco seasoning.
- Cook until sweet potatoes are tender. Serve with a dollop of Greek yogurt.

Nutritional Value:

- Protein: 25g
- Carbohydrates: 30g
- Fats: 8g

Grilled Turkey Burgers

Prep Time: 20 minutes

Ingredients:

- 1 lb ground turkey
- Whole grain burger buns
- Lettuce, tomato, and red onion
- Your favorite condiments

Instructions:

- Form turkey into patties, grill until fully cooked.
- Assemble burgers with your preferred toppings. Enjoy with a side salad.

Nutritional Value:

- Protein: 25g
- Carbohydrates: 30g
- Fats: 10g

Lemon Garlic Roast Chicken

Prep Time: 15 minutes

Ingredients:

- Whole roasting chicken
- Zest and juice of 2 lemons
- Garlic cloves, minced
- Fresh rosemary and thyme

Instructions:

- Preheat oven. Rub chicken with lemon zest, juice, garlic, and herbs.
- Roast until golden and fully cooked. Serve with roasted vegetables.

Nutritional Value:

- Protein: 30g
- Carbohydrates: 1g
- Fats: 15g

Turkey and Black Bean Chili

Prep Time: 30 minutes

Ingredients:

- 1 lb ground turkey
- 1 can black beans, drained
- Diced tomatoes, onion, and bell peppers
- Chili powder, cumin, and paprika

Instructions:

- Brown turkey, add beans, tomatoes, vegetables, and spices.
- Simmer until flavors meld. Serve with a dollop of Greek yogurt.

Nutritional Value:

- Protein: 25g
- Carbohydrates: 30g
- Fats: 8g

Chicken and Broccoli Quinoa Bowl

Prep Time: 25 minutes

Ingredients:

- 1 lb chicken breast, cubed
- Broccoli florets
- Cooked quinoa
- Soy sauce, ginger, and garlic

Instructions:

- Stirfry chicken and broccoli in a pan with soy sauce, ginger, and garlic.
- Serve over a bed of quinoa. A well-balanced and satisfying meal.

Nutritional Value:

- Protein: 30g
- Carbohydrates: 30g
- Fats: 8g

These chicken and turkey recipes are tailored for a macro diet, providing a delicious and protein-packed foundation for your balanced nutrition.

31-Day Macro Diet Meal Plan

Day 1

Breakfast: Greek Yogurt and Berry Parfait

Lunch: Grilled Lemon Herb Chicken Breast with Quinoa

Dinner: Baked Pesto Salmon with Roasted Vegetables

Day 2

Breakfast: Protein-Packed Chocolate Smoothie Bowl

Lunch: Turkey and Quinoa Stuffed Peppers

Dinner: Chicken and Broccoli Quinoa Bowl

Day 3

Breakfast: Avocado Toast with Poached Eggs

Lunch: Chickpea and Vegetable Stir-Fry

Dinner: Lemon Garlic Roast Chicken with Sweet Potato Mash

Day 4

Breakfast: Whole Grain Oatmeal with Berries and Almond Butter

Lunch: Caprese Salad with Grilled Chicken

Dinner: Turkey and Sweet Potato Skillet

Day 5

Breakfast: Scrambled Eggs with Spinach and Feta

Lunch: Baked Pesto Chicken Thighs with Quinoa

Dinner: Grilled Turkey Burgers with Mixed Greens Salad

Day 6

Breakfast: Chia Seed Pudding with Mixed Berries

Lunch: Chicken and Spinach Stuffed Portobello Mushrooms

Dinner: Grilled Lemon Herb Shrimp Skewers with Brown Rice

Day 7

Breakfast: Banana and Almond Butter Smoothie

Lunch: Turkey and Black Bean Chili

Dinner: Baked Cod with Asparagus and Quinoa

Day 8

Breakfast: Mango and Coconut Yogurt Parfait

Lunch: Grilled Chicken Caesar Salad with Whole Grain Croutons

Dinner: Turkey and Vegetable Skewers with Quinoa

Day 9

Breakfast: Overnight Oats with Sliced Peaches and Almonds

Lunch: Mediterranean Chickpea Salad with Feta

Dinner: Baked Lemon Herb Tilapia with Broccoli and Brown Rice

Day 10

Breakfast: Protein Pancakes with Fresh Berries

Lunch: Turkey and Avocado Wrap with Whole Wheat Tortilla

Dinner: Chicken and Vegetable Curry with Cauliflower Rice

Day 11

Breakfast: Egg White Omelette with Spinach and Tomatoes

Lunch: Quinoa and Black Bean Bowl with Grilled Chicken

Dinner: Salmon and Asparagus Foil Packets with Lemon Dill Sauce

Day 12

Breakfast: Blueberry and Almond Butter Smoothie Bowl

Lunch: Greek Chicken Souvlaki Salad

Dinner: Turkey Meatballs with Zucchini Noodles and Marinara Sauce

Day 13

Breakfast: Cottage Cheese with Pineapple and Walnuts

Lunch: Chickpea and Avocado Salad

Dinner: Grilled Shrimp and Vegetable StirFry with Brown Rice

Day 14

Breakfast: Banana Nut Protein Muffins

Lunch: Turkey and Hummus Wrap with Whole Wheat Pita

Dinner: Baked Chicken Thighs with Brussels Sprouts and Quinoa

Day 15

Breakfast: Protein Waffles with Mixed Berry Compote

Lunch: Lentil and Vegetable Soup with Grilled Chicken Salad

Dinner: Baked Cod with Mango Salsa and Quinoa

Day 16

Breakfast: Avocado and Bacon Breakfast Burrito

Lunch: Turkey and Vegetable Skewers with Tzatziki Sauce

Dinner: Lemon Herb Grilled Tofu with Roasted Vegetables

Day 17

Breakfast: Chocolate Banana Protein Smoothie

Lunch: Quinoa Salad with Roasted Veggies and Feta

Dinner: Chicken Fajita Bowl with Brown Rice

Day 18

Breakfast: Overnight Chia Seed Pudding with Kiwi and Coconut

Lunch: Greek Turkey Burger with Greek Salad

Dinner: Baked Salmon with Herbed Quinoa

Day 19

Breakfast: Spinach and Mushroom Egg White Scramble

Lunch: Chickpea and Spinach Curry with Cauliflower Rice

Dinner: Turkey Taco Bowl with Black Beans and Salsa

Day 20

Breakfast: Peanut Butter Banana Protein Muffins

Lunch: Grilled Chicken and Vegetable Wrap with Hummus

Dinner: Shrimp and Avocado Salad with Lime Vinaigrette

Day 21

Breakfast: Mango Coconut Chia Pudding

Lunch: Turkey and Quinoa Stuffed Acorn Squash

Dinner: Baked Lemon Herb Halibut with Asparagus

Day 22

Breakfast: Blueberry Almond Protein Smoothie Bowl

Lunch: Quinoa and Black Bean Stuffed Bell Peppers

Dinner: Grilled Tofu Skewers with Peanut Sauce and Brown Rice

Day 23

Breakfast: Cottage Cheese Pancakes with Strawberry Compote

Lunch: Turkey and Hummus Veggie Wrap

Dinner: Baked Chicken Breast with Lemon Dill Sauce and Steamed Broccoli

Day 24

Breakfast: Protein-Packed Breakfast Burrito with Salsa

Lunch: Lentil and Chickpea Salad with Grilled Chicken

Dinner: Baked Cod with Tomato and Olive Relish and Quinoa

Day 25

Breakfast: Banana Walnut Overnight Oats

Lunch: Turkey and Vegetable Stir-Fry with Brown Rice

Dinner: Grilled Shrimp Tacos with Cabbage Slaw

Day 26

Breakfast: Scrambled Eggs with Spinach and Feta

Lunch: Greek Chicken Souvlaki Bowl with Tzatziki

Dinner: Baked Salmon with Mango Avocado Salsa and Sweet Potato

Day 27

Breakfast: Protein-Packed Blueberry Muffins

Lunch: Quinoa Salad with Roasted Vegetables and Grilled Chicken

Dinner: Chicken and Vegetable Curry with Cauliflower Rice

Day 28

Breakfast: Peanut Butter Banana Protein Smoothie

Lunch: Turkey and Quinoa Stuffed Zucchini Boats

Dinner: Lemon Herb Grilled Tofu with Asparagus and Quinoa

Day 29

Breakfast: Almond Butter and Banana Protein Pancakes

Lunch: Chickpea and Avocado Salad with Grilled Chicken

Dinner: Baked Lemon Herb Halibut with Roasted Brussels Sprouts

Day 30

Breakfast: Chocolate Protein Chia Seed Pudding

Lunch: Turkey and Sweet Potato Skillet

Dinner: Grilled Shrimp and Vegetable Kabobs with Quinoa

Day 31

Breakfast: Mixed Berry and Almond Butter Smoothie Bowl

Lunch: Chicken Caesar Salad with Whole Grain Croutons

Dinner: Baked Cod with Mediterranean Quinoa

This completes your 31day Macro Diet meal plan. Remember to stay hydrated with water, incorporate snacks like nuts or Greek yogurt as needed, and listen to your body's hunger and fullness cues. Feel free to repeat

your favorite meals or introduce new recipes to keep your

diet diverse and enjoyable. The Macro Diet is all about

flexibility and sustainability, so adapt this plan to suit your

individual preferences and nutritional needs. Enjoy your

journey towards a healthier and more balanced lifestyle!

Intermittent Fasting (IF)

The goal of the eating pattern known as Intermittent Fasting (IF) is to optimize health and promote weight management by alternating between periods of eating and fasting. In this method, the timing of meals is more important than the kinds of foods eaten. Different forms of intermittent fasting allow people more leeway to tailor the plan to their own tastes and routines by establishing different times for fasting and eating.

When to Fast:

In the 16/8 Method, you fast for 16 hours every day and then eat within an 8-hour window.

In the 18/6 Method, which is comparable to the 16/8 Method, the fasting period is 18 hours rather than 8 and the eating window is 6 hours rather than 8.

On the 5:2 diet, you eat normally five days a week and drastically cut back (by 500 to 600 calories) on two days that aren't consecutive.

Advantages

Weight Management: As IF limits the eating window, calorie intake is lowered, which may help with weight loss.

Enhanced Metabolism: by increasing fat oxidation and enhancing insulin sensitivity, IF may improve metabolic health, according to some research.

Fasting triggers autophagy, a cellular repair mechanism that involves removing damaged cells and replacing them with new, healthy ones.

Brain Health: IF may promote cognitive function and protect against neurodegenerative disorders by boosting the production of brain-derived neurotrophic factor (BDNF).

Getting Started

Choose an approach: Select an IF approach that corresponds with your lifestyle and tastes.

Stay Hydrated: Drink plenty of water, herbal teas, and black coffee during fasting periods.

Balanced Nutrition: Focus on nutrient-dense meals when eating, ensuring you meet your nutritional demands.

Listen to Your Body: Pay attention to hunger cues and modify fasting windows accordingly.

Considerations

Individual Variability: The effectiveness of IF can differ among individuals. Some people may find it easier to adhere to, while others may have difficulty.

Health issues: Individuals with specific health issues, such as diabetes or eating disorders, should consult a healthcare expert before starting IF.

Consistency: Consistency is crucial for long-term success with IF. Establish a schedule that fits your lifestyle.

Caution

Not Suitable for Everyone: Pregnant or breastfeeding women, persons with a history of eating problems, and those with specific medical conditions should avoid IF or perform it under strong medical supervision.

Potential Side Effects: Some people may feel irritation, weariness, or difficulty concentrating, especially during the early transition phase.

Intermittent Fasting can be an effective and adaptable technique for weight management and overall health enhancement. However, it's vital to approach it wisely, considering individual needs and potential health effects. Consulting with a healthcare professional or nutritionist before starting an Intermittent Fasting regimen is advisable to ensure it aligns with your unique health profile.

Ketogenic Diet

The Ketogenic Diet, commonly known as the Keto Diet, is a low-carbohydrate, high-fat eating plan designed to produce a state of ketosis in the body. In ketosis, the body shifts from using glucose as its primary energy source to burning fats for fuel. This metabolic state has garnered attention for its potential benefits in weight loss, improved mental clarity, and increased energy levels.

Macronutrient Composition

- **High Fat:** Approximately 70-75% of daily caloric intake comes from healthy fats such as avocados, nuts, seeds, and oils.

- **Moderate Protein:** Protein intake is moderate, comprising about 20-25% of daily calories.

- **Low Carbohydrate:** Carbohydrates are severely restricted, typically accounting for only 5-10% of daily caloric intake.

Ketosis

By minimizing carbohydrate intake, the body depletes its glycogen stores and enters a state of ketosis. - In ketosis, the liver produces ketones from fats, which become the primary source of energy for the body and brain.

Food Choices

- **Healthy Fats:** Avocados, olive oil, coconut oil, nuts, seeds, and fatty fish.

- **Moderate Proteins:** Poultry, fish, meat, eggs, and dairy products.

Low Carbohydrates: Leafy green vegetables, non-starchy vegetables, and minimal whole grains.

Benefits

- **Weight Loss:** The Keto Diet is effective for weight loss, primarily due to reduced carbohydrate intake leading to lower insulin levels and increased fat burning.

- **Improved Mental Clarity:** Some individuals report enhanced cognitive function and mental clarity in ketosis.

- **Stabilized Blood Sugar:** The diet may help stabilize blood sugar levels, beneficial for individuals with insulin resistance.

Potential Challenges

- **Keto Flu:** During the initial adaption phase, individuals may experience symptoms including weariness, headaches, and irritability, together known as the "Keto flu."

- **Nutrient shortages:** Severely reducing some food groups can lead to nutrient shortages, thus cautious planning is important.

Health Considerations

- Consultation with Healthcare specialists: Individuals with pre-existing health concerns, especially those connected to the heart, liver, or kidneys, should speak with healthcare specialists before commencing the Keto Diet.

- Individual Variability: The effectiveness of the Keto Diet can differ among individuals. Some may thrive on it, while others may find it tough to maintain.

Sustainability

Lifestyle Commitment: The Keto Diet needs a major commitment to reducing carbohydrates, making it vital to analyze its sustainability for individual lifestyles.

Cyclical Ketogenic Diet (CKD)

Some individuals follow a CKD, which entails cycling between periods of strict ketosis and greater carbohydrate intake.

The Keto Diet can be an effective tool for weight loss and certain health benefits, but it's vital to approach it wisely. Consulting with healthcare specialists or nutritionists before commencing the Keto Diet is suggested, especially for people with underlying health concerns. Additionally, following the diet with a focus on nutrient-dense, whole foods ensures a more balanced approach to long-term health and well-being.

Conclusion

In closing this detailed guide to the Macro Diet Cookbook for Beginners, it's apparent that taking a balanced and flexible approach to eating may be a transforming journey towards increased health and wellbeing. Throughout the book, we've explored the fundamental concepts of macro dieting, gone into the nuances of macronutrients—proteins, carbs, and fats—and presented a vast array of dishes geared for newcomers on this culinary voyage.

The Macro Diet, with its emphasis on customization and individualization, exceeds traditional concepts of dieting. It's not just about counting calories; it's about understanding and maximizing the nutritional makeup of what we consume. The versatility of this method permits individuals to achieve varied health and fitness goals, from weight management to muscle building, all while cultivating a positive connection with food.

Our investigation of the Macro Diet journey covers not just the basics of macro tracking but also delved into the art of defining personalized macro goals. Understanding the value of proteins, carbs, and fats allows us to adjust nutrition to individual needs, establishing a blueprint for prolonged energy, increased performance, and overall vitality.

The benefits of macro dieting extend far beyond the domain of physical health. By increasing attention regarding food choices and portion sizes, the Macro Diet offers a holistic approach to nutrition. The recipes featured in this cookbook highlight the amazing possibilities within macro-friendly meals, emphasizing that a balanced diet should not sacrifice flavor or diversity.

Furthermore, we've shown the flexibility of the Macro Diet to varied dietary choices. Whether you're a meat lover, a vegetarian, or following to special dietary restrictions, the Macro Diet supports a broad spectrum of eating choices, assuring inclusion and accessibility.

As we complete the chapters of this Macro Diet Cookbook for Beginners, we welcome you to embark on a culinary trip that goes beyond the typical confines of dieting. Embrace the freedom to choose foods that resonate with your taste buds, while aligning with your health and fitness objectives. May this cookbook serve as a beneficial resource, helping you to traverse the world of macronutrients and make tasty, macro-friendly meals that nourish both body and soul. Here's to your health, wellness, and the unlimited possibilities that the Macro Diet may bring to your table. Happy cooking!

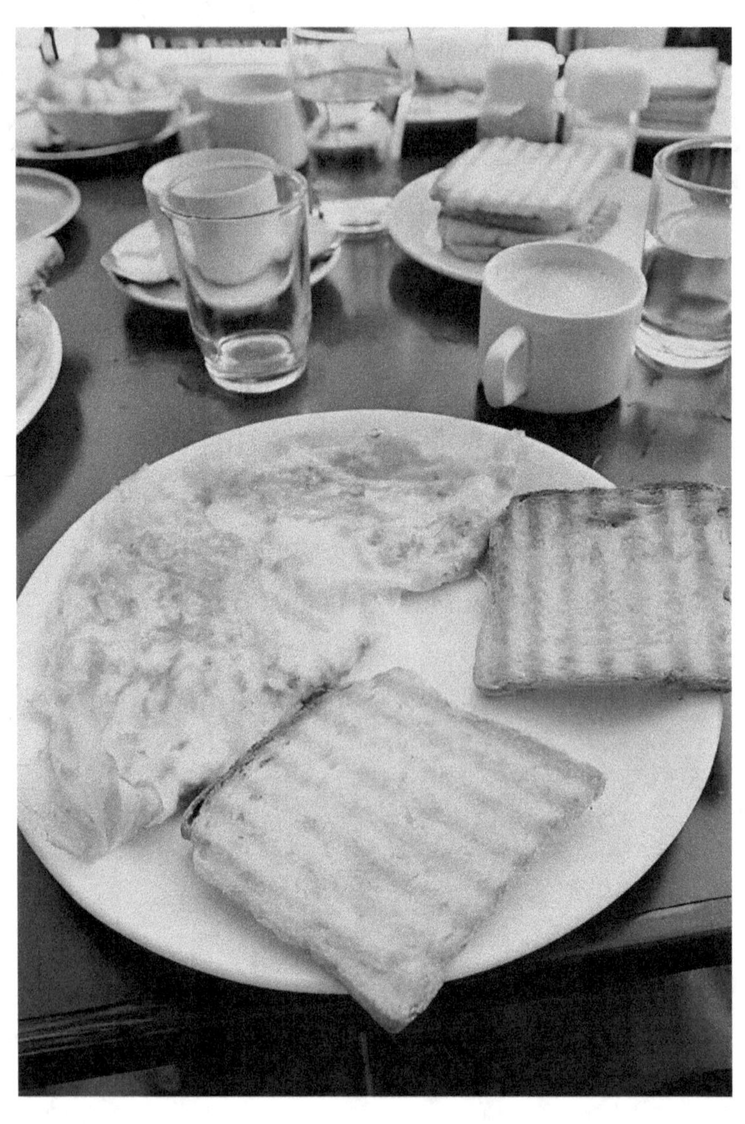